The Healing Call of Cancer

Sue Paulson

Published by FingerTip Solutions, 2024.

THE HEALING CALL OF CANCER

First edition. October 15, 2024.

Written by Sue Paulson.

Table of Contents

Chapter 1 | Diagnosis Day 1

Chapter 2 | Focus on the Physical 9

Chapter 3 | You & Your Healing Team 19

Chapter 4 | The Process of Treatment 27

Chapter 5 | Exploring Thoughts & Feelings 41

Chapter 6 | Exploring & Changing Our Minds.......................51

Chapter 7 | Thoughts Become Things...57

Chapter 8 | A Trip to Heaven..69

Chapter 9 | You -Creator of Your Own Reality 77

To all the courageous Souls whose lives cancer has touched.
Bless you, everyone!

The Offering

The goal of this book is to support cancer sufferers and their loved ones as they face one of life's most challenging journeys. Cancer doesn't affect only the sufferers. It affects all of us. This book is about the human side of cancer, not only its challenges, but the triumphs and gifts that can emerge.

Having survived cancer twice, I'm not only still standing, but I have been thriving for the past twelve years. Despite a persistent voice that poked, prodded, and pushed, I was resistant to writing anything more about cancer after my first book, *Magnificent Misery – From Adversity to Ecstasy* was released in 2015. Then my sister got cancer and died at age 50 in 2021. So I picked up my pen again.

Being neither a medical professional nor a cancer researcher, I have only written about what I've observed and learned from my own experience and the experiences of others.

Perhaps you're like me, with biases for and against certain things. Any opinions expressed are mine alone. For example:

Because I look for the good in everything, I believe there are gifts in and even from the darkest of life's moments. Some call me the quintessential Pollyanna. I confess, that's me.

I do not believe that cancer happens randomly to people – there is a reason – a good reason that you got it, and I got it. It didn't come from outside our bodies like an enemy invader. We all have cancer cells in our bodies. Usually, our immune systems eliminate them, or they die off on their own. But when they grow or cluster, it's a signal that something much bigger is going on.

Why any of it happens is still a mystery to me. But I do believe that cancer is **not** the enemy. It is, however, a formidable teacher. Cancer has much to teach us about ourselves, our lives, and about the world we live in. You may or may not figure out why you and cancer became acquainted. But I promise you, if you look, there will be gifts arising from this adversity.

The way I chose to heal is not the only way. If something I say doesn't resonate with you, set it aside and keep searching for what feels right for you. There are many books, internet articles, professionals, and the experiences of others that you can reference.

My fondest wish is that you, my readers, will find lifelines, tools, and/or rays of hope to assist you on this path, not only through cancer but to a magnificent life beyond.

I honor each of you in your quest for healing.

Sue Paulson

Cancer and Me ©

This cancer has hollowed me out.

Stripped me of the bones of everything I ever

knew, was, or thought I could be.

Who am I now

with the specter of death

hovering so near?

I seek my old self

and find but echoes

of a life I believed

was well-lived.

How do I proceed?

Can I create anew,

or will life's uncertainty

stop me in my tracks?

Will Fear be the victor?

INTRODUCTION

Cancer has called you. Here you are, face to face.

The great unknown beckons – to what you don't yet know. But you have been here before – on the precipice of some other kind of adversity. Remember how you were stronger than all those other adversities? Though it might not feel like it, you are stronger now – stronger than this terror, and stronger than this cancer. In my bones, I know that you are strong enough to go head-to-head with it.

Likely this cancer feels like the enemy – the enemy that could kill you. No wonder you're scared! In 2011, I stood in the same spot as you when cancer called; I felt the same terror. You need to know you are not alone.

Let me be clear. I don't have a "cure". I don't have The Answer. What I have are thoughts, experiences, suggestions, and guidance that may help you on this healing journey. This book is about You. Take what feels right – what resonates with you – and leave the rest.

I've taken a holistic approach which, along with the body, includes mind, emotions, and spirit. I've come to understand that while the initial focus to eradicate cancer cells is often only centered on the physical body, full healing comes from an intense focus on our mental and emotional states and the condition of our spirit. It will take the holy trinity of YOU to not only survive cancer, but to thrive beyond it.

Rather than seeing cancer as a failure of some kind (what I did wrong, what I didn't do, this is a punishment, I'm to blame) consider that cancer has arrived in your life to become your teacher, your catalyst – your wake-up call. Like it or not, life often tests us first – learning comes later. For some of you, it's an opportunity to heal all of you in order to live life more fully than ever before. For others, along with healing, it's your path to shed the body and take that final journey Home.

First, let's face the fact that our physical bodies are going to die of something, right? While we never know what will take us out or when that will happen, right now, death is inevitable.

But even if you can't know for sure whether this cancer will kill you or you will kill it, you are alive in this moment. Why not choose to live your life to its fullest regardless of the amount of time you have left?

My experience of cancer gave me an opportunity to end previous suffering and learn to live a most joyful life – in fact, heaven on earth. I want that for you!

Regardless of your ultimate destination, this is a complex journey. As with any hero's quest, you have some inherent power tools to support you:

Courage

Determination

Faith

Hope

- **Courage**: In the face of fear, we can call upon our reserves of courage – we can even lean on others and borrow their courage. At times, you will feel vulnerable. That's good. According to Brene Brown, there is no courage without vulnerability. Small acts of bravery can fuel your courage.
- **Determination**: Humans are hard-wired to overcome adversity. When the going gets rough, we dig a little deeper for the energy to keep going, no matter how hard it gets.
- **Faith**: Faith can move mountains. If you are a religious or spiritual person, your faith in a higher power is a mighty tool. Even if you have no religious beliefs, faith still exists - faith in yourself and the faith of your loved ones -all at your disposal.

You are not alone!

- **Hope**: Hope is defined as a feeling of trust – a feeling of expectation and desire for certain things to happen. When we build and maintain our hope for the best outcome, it sustains us through the darkest of times. *(Anatomy of Hope – How People Prevail in the Face of Illness, Jerome Groopman, M.D.)*

While none of these power tools can be seen or scientifically measured, collectively they make you tougher than any cancer. When you combine them with whatever treatment protocol you choose, you improve your chances of moving beyond cancer.

Chapter 1
Diagnosis Day

"Cancer is a word, not a sentence." John Diamond

When you get a cancer diagnosis, you cannot unhear the words that pronounce the verdict. You cannot unsee any pictures they've shown you - where the cancer is and how big it is. This is a major turning point in your life. Because of this news, nothing is going to be the same. Much as you want to, you cannot turn back to your old life. You can only turn to face an unknown and uncertain future.

I remember that day in February 2011 when the doctor showed me the graphic pictures of the tumor near my rectum and confirmed I had cancer. To say I was shocked and horrified is an understatement. Likely you felt something similar receiving your diagnosis.

The Pit of Denial

Elizabeth Kubler-Ross, who wrote the book, *On Death and Dying* listed the first stage of grief as denial. The shock that comes from a traumatic diagnosis can certainly drop you into the pit of denial. Questions pop up in the mind:

How could this happen to me? What have I done wrong? Is this a punishment? Why Me?

It's quickly followed by a myriad of thoughts:

This cannot be happening. This isn't fair. I'm a good person. I didn't do anything to deserve this. Maybe the diagnosis is wrong. I feel fine.

Fear, anger, numbness, sadness – our emotions and our thoughts are all over the map.

THE HEALING CALL OF CANCER

Naturally, in those moments, no one is ready to face the reality of their diagnosis. And yet, to move forward, it's important to find a way out of the pit toward acceptance – even if it's acceptance of the smallest piece of this news. You don't have to like it, but facing this reality will help you deal with whatever's in front of you.

Of course, everyone moves in and out of denial and in and out of acceptance at his or her own pace. I certainly did. It took me a long time to work through it – I was in denial about being in denial!

One way to come to terms with this news is by making two lists: First, what you believe is "bad" about having cancer and, second, any possible blessings in having cancer. Your first list might include the following points:

- It could kill me.
- I could lose my job.
- My spouse might leave me.
- My kids will be left alone.
- I will die without having really lived.
- I can't afford treatment.

Now the second list - finding blessings - might seem impossible at this stage. And that's o.k. Create the sheet anyway for future use. Many of my blessings showed up later.

It was fascinating to me how survivors told me that cancer was the best thing that ever happened to them. Initial blessings might be things such as

- People will stop expecting so much from me.
- I can stop doing the job I've disliked for so many years.
- I can shift my attention to me and my healing.
- Once I get through cancer, I can choose a new life based on

what I most love.

It isn't what's on the list that's important. The result of focusing in a logical way on this new problem takes you out of denial for a few moments so your mind can begin to process what is happening. Just remember that solutions are hard to find when we deny there's a problem.

William Bridges talks about the difference between change and transition. As we know, situations can change in a heartbeat. But in order for us to transition through any change, we need time for our brains, minds, and hearts to move from denial through to acceptance.

My dear sister initially viewed her stage 4 diagnosis as merely a chronic condition. She wouldn't fully acknowledge or talk about it for at least a year. Why? Her fear of dying young was so opposite to her vision for her life and what she had yet to accomplish, that her brain refused to come to grips with the new reality.

During your struggle to process and ultimately accept what's happening, find as much compassion for yourself as you can muster. Everyone's journey is different. You will work through this in your own way and in your own time – one piece at a time is o.k. Surround yourself with compassionate people you feel comfortable sharing with. Or if there's no one there for you, get a journal and work through things on paper.

The other stages of grief leading to acceptance include anger, bargaining, and depression. It's **normal** to bounce back and forth in random order, or even skip a stage. There is no "right" way to deal with this kind of news. Resist the urge to compare your progress to anyone else. Where you are is where you are, and that's as it should be.

Questions to Ponder after Diagnosis

- How will my life change?
- Who will I share this diagnosis with?
- Who can I count on for support?
- What do I need to do to prepare for what comes next?
- Although I have cancer, does it define who I really am?
- Am I more powerful than this cancer?

Research

Our feelings hardly settle down before the oncologists and other professionals step in with their recommended repertoire of treatments and tools. In order for them to do battle with your cancer, their goal is to get you scheduled as quickly as possible – "Here's the plan – now let's get you booked."

Before you say yes to anything, if you can, buy yourself some time.

You know how financial advisors suggest that you take time away when you have a big lottery win – just so you can adjust to the impact of how your life will change? I recommend the same thing here. While this situation may seem more like a "loser lottery" in the wheel of fortune, the enormity of the change is similar. It's important to give yourself precious time, either alone or with loved ones. Step back and take a deep breath.

Resist the urge to instantly succumb to the medical merry-go-round until you're good and ready – trust me, it's not so merry. Even if a life-threatening situation sent you for emergency surgery and you didn't have the opportunity to absorb what was happening, you have time before whatever comes next; you need that time:

- To adjust mentally and emotionally

- To research
- To gather your supporters
- To decide about your next course of action

This is your body and your life. Regardless of what the professionals want, you have both the right and the responsibility to decide the next step.

Right after my diagnosis, my mate went into research mode not only about my cancer, but about the various recommended treatment protocols and their side effects.

While he was doing that, I searched for survivor stories. I needed to know that it was possible for me to live through this. I read and heard plenty of stories both on and offline that gave me hope. Encouraging, too, were the overall stats I found about cancer – mortality rates for most types of cancer have been steadily dropping since 1985.

All this research was focused on the physical aspect of my well-being but not it's root cause. (Some medical professionals believe that the mind, body, and spirit are sick long before cancer shows up as a symptom. According to prominent researchers, chronic stress (dis-ease) is a key contributor to every major illness, including cancer. More about this in later chapters.)

When it comes to treatment protocols, don't be surprised by the overwhelm you may feel as you sift through descriptions and side effects. I was horrified when surgery and its devastating result was described. I was also terrified when I read about the doctors' recommended route of chemo and radiation.

Making Decisions

Once you have the information you need, your job is to pick what feels right based on your diagnosis and life circumstances.

As an example, because I suspected that my body was not healthy enough initially to survive the doctors' prescribed treatment, I chose a more holistic, alternative healing camp in order to get strong.

In my 30s, I had had success with various methods for other health challenges. Despite the high cost of them (and no medical coverage) the treatments were far less invasive or debilitating, plus I liked the fact that they were designed to support the body's own ability to heal.

Along with your chosen treatments, be sure that the professionals you meet are open to hearing your concerns and ideas. That openness and their listening ability is important so you can develop a high level of trust with them. These people will help you manage your treatment and care and support you in staying in your own power.

While you may not be a cancer expert, you are the one most familiar with your own mind, body, and soul. You are the decision maker, and that's as it should be. Will what you pick work? No guarantees, of course. What I know for sure - if it's not your time to go, nothing will kill you. If it is your time to go, no treatment will work to "save" your life. In the meantime, you have decisions to make.

An important side note here: If your cancer is a virulent kind and you're told you have a short time to live, please **don't panic!** Doctors work with statistics, probabilities, and historical information that they have so far. Although their stats provide some information, they cannot factor in the uniqueness of every individual. One cousin of mine, with an initial Stage 4 breast cancer diagnosis and a predicted short time to live lasted over 11 years.

Remember I mentioned hope, faith, courage, and determination – essential components to healing? There are plenty of anecdotes that support how powerful those tools are. One inspiring story is Anita Moorjani's book, *Dying to Be Me*.

Regardless of your kind of cancer, **you** are your best chance of survival.

Chapter 2
Focus on the Physical

"Yesterday is gone, tomorrow has not come. We have only today. Let us begin." **Mother Teresa**

Body Signals

Whether it's pain and discomfort or a sense of aliveness and well-being, our bodies are magnificent at communicating what's working and what's not.

Just as we start noticing the world around us through our senses when we're born, our bodies also send signals to us all the time about how everything is functioning or not functioning.

Signals of hunger, discomfort, pain, or tiredness come through automatically. When the problem is dealt with, the signals stop. Our bodies are miraculous enough that even when we ignore pain or discomfort, they keep functioning, sometimes for years.

I ignored my body's signals far too long. Constipation, blood in my stool, hemorrhoids, embarrassing halitosis – each telling me to get checked out. By the time I acted, it was too late for a simple treatment. Cancer cells had clustered into an undeniable mass that would prove tough to eradicate.

Even in the face of a traumatic diagnosis, I clung to the idea that I must continue with my life, regardless. "Soldiering on" was ingrained in me. People were counting on me. I was not about to stop for cancer! (Here's my denial, right here.)

How might our lives be different if we paid attention to those little warnings? Because really – where are you going to live when your body gives out? We can create our own brand of hell on earth simply by refusing to treat our bodies as the sacred vessels that they are.

My Choices After Diagnosis

In my situation, I said no initially to the proposed radiation and chemo protocol. Why? The first reason - the condescending attitude of the oncologist ticked me off when he scoffed at my ideas and wouldn't listen to me. Secondly, at the time of diagnosis, I wasn't in the best shape physically.

So, I bought myself some time, not only to come to terms with the diagnosis, but to focus on the overall health of the rest of my body. Of course, once I turned my back on the cancer institute, the door slammed shut - I was on my own.

Through trial and error and bravado mixed with fear, I chose a blend of naturopathic and natural remedies. I first visited a practitioner who conducted live blood cell analysis and then recommended a strict food protocol that eliminated most grains, dairy, sugar, and most meats. Initially, I was allowed a limited amount of fruit and encouraged to eat plenty of vegetables. The weight dropped off, I had more energy, and I started to feel much better.

My frantic, naive search for my own *magic bullet* to cure me led to some weird protocols that were neither scientifically proven nor effective. I tried, unsuccessfully, to manage my treatment. There were just too many components to a complex situation, including my erratic emotions. I made costly mistakes, but I learned. Fortunately for me I survived being my own guinea pig!

During those six months, what supported me most was a consistent series of intravenous vitamin C dosages administered by a skilled naturopath who specialized in working with cancer patients. Both the altered diet and the vitamin C regime were successful in getting me to a strong and healthy state. What it didn't do was reduce my tumor. A subsequent MRI, ordered by my family doctor at my request showed increased tumor growth.

Reluctantly, I went back to the cancer institute (to a different oncologist). According to their stats, the radiation-chemo combo for my cancer was supposed to deliver a "cure"– 73% chance – quite good odds, I thought.

In reality, the third round of chemo nearly killed me, and radiation caused severe pain, nasty groin burns, and an extremely unreliable bowel. Instead of the anticipated cure, their treatment eliminated the tumor for only six months.

When the tumor came back in the same spot, radical surgery was my only option. I continued high and frequent doses of intravenous Vitamin C to help me through the worst of it.

It was strange that both the oncologist and the surgeon commented about me doing much better than all their other patients. Yet they never asked what I was doing differently – and I never volunteered. I guess I was too scared of repercussions!

Battling through two bouts of cancer has a way of shifting one's focus. Others experience heart attacks, strokes, broken bones, "accidents" and other debilitating conditions. If you track back, there were tiny physical signals long before the big event.

THE HEALING CALL OF CANCER

There's a great little book by Spencer Johnson called, *One Minute for Myself.* He encourages readers to ask themselves, "Is there a better way I can take care of myself right now?" Cancer is one way of waking us up to focus on what our bodies need from us.

A cancer diagnosis commands our attention and our respect. Remember though, the body is not like a car that we take to the mechanic for fixing. The major pain of car repairs is paying the bill. The body, however, is inextricably linked with feelings and thoughts. While our physical well-being is at stake, the diagnosis also triggers a deep primal fear because of its life-threatening nature.

Fear will be a constant companion along with any choice you make - that's a natural reaction – you're human. It's vital though that you don't allow fear to hold you hostage and dictate your choices because of moments of panic.

I know, and I hope you will come to know that you are not only stronger than cancer; you are stronger than your fear. Can you love yourself enough to set aside or work through unreasoning fear? Strange as it may seem, love, particularly self-love is the antidote to fear.

Love yourself enough to take time to breathe. Please breathe until you feel a moment of calm. Regardless of your diagnosis, you have time. There will be many decisions regarding treatment and healing that are yours to make.

While you may not feel in control of your cancer and this situation, **you are in charge**. You have the right and the power to say yes or no to any treatment proposed. You are also responsible for the outcomes of your choices.

Let me provide my simplistic understanding of the two schools of thought regarding cancer treatment:

1. **The Western Allopathic Medicine Approach:** Cancer is the enemy in the body, so the task is to radiate, poison, and/or cut out the cells – whatever the cost to the immune system or healthy cells in the rest of the body. The goal has always been to kill cancer cells in order to save/prolong the patient's life. Death is the enemy which doctors and oncologists fight against.

Improvements to radiation equipment have helped reduce the slaughter of healthy cells. Plus, there are more sophisticated chemo cocktails for specific cancers.

Despite these advances, research shows that chemo and radiation only kill cancer cells temporarily. Lifespan increase is mere months instead of the years that were hoped for.

Even though public statements about ineffectiveness have been made by trusted cancer researchers over the past several years, these treatments are still the standard, approved protocol.

1. **The Complementary/Alternative Therapies Approach:** The human body is a self-healing organism with an army of immune fighters capable of killing cancer cells. When the body is supported with non-toxic therapies and supplements, the immune system is boosted, and the body can do the job it was designed for.

There is plenty of anecdotal evidence to point to success and failure rates but only a small sampling of peer-reviewed studies due to the lack of research funds.

THE HEALING CALL OF CANCER

Let me emphasize that neither of these camps has found a "cure" for cancer. Some people die from cancer, and some people live, despite cancer.

NOTE: Travis Christofferson's *Tripping Over the Truth: The Return of the Metabolic Theory of Cancer Illuminates a New and Hopeful Path to a Cure* is a worthwhile read. It documents the journey of cancer research – the good, the bad, and the ugly. The author is a medical research doctor who was curious about treating cancer in less invasive ways.

Along with the "war" on cancer, there are many skirmishes between both of the above camps. The Allopathic Camp still continues to warn patients about trying anything outside of their own protocol. However, that approach is shifting as some oncologists, having seen benefits particularly from therapies out of Germany, are quietly supportive of certain complementary disciplines.

Patients who use any alternative treatments rarely share that with their oncologists for fear of repercussions. I was fortunate to have a Naturopath who had been a pharmacist. He knew what supplements would safeguard me from the harm of the chemo drugs I was using.

I long for the day when health professionals from all arenas cooperate and collaborate for the ultimate good of their patients. The territorialism serves only to make the drug companies richer. (Sorry, my bias has raised its head here – hence the political comment!)

With ingrained beliefs that their doctors know best, many cancer patients turn themselves over to the western cancer clinics to be "fixed". Your families, who also feel terrified by your diagnosis, may urge you to do whatever the doctors say, no questions asked.

Two doctors said to me, "Well, if you were my mother, I would want you to have this treatment." In the face of all that pressure, it's easy to ignore questions about the cost or collateral damage to our bodies from certain treatments.

I know too many cancer patients who later felt betrayed by doctors who weren't candid about potential harm to their bodies because of chemo or radiation. These patients also didn't know what questions to ask.

To help you make an informed decision, here are some questions to get you started:

- What are the most common risks associated with the proposed treatment?
- Will I be able to work while undergoing treatment?
- How much of my treatment is covered by insurance?
- How will you help me manage any pain?
- What happens if I don't respond well to the course of treatment?
- What are the long-term effects of treatment on the rest of my body?
- How will the disease progress if I refuse treatment?

Depending on your age and/or stage of life and your stage of cancer, it's important to consider not just the quantity but your quality of life.

For example, the father of a dear friend who was diagnosed with lung cancer in his 80s, having previously witnessed his wife's suffering from chemo and radiation to treat her lung cancer, refused recommended treatment. He chose to have doctors and family help him manage his pain in the comfort of his own home.

THE HEALING CALL OF CANCER

My sister was in her mid-40s when diagnosed with stage 4 of a rare cancer. A business owner and single mom of a teenage son, she allowed experimental "hail Mary" treatments and fought through horrific side effects to be there for her son as long as possible.

As sad as we were when she died at age 50, it was a relief to have her no longer suffering. No one can really know if her decisions were the "right" ones, but they were hers to make.

Knowing what I'd discovered about chemo and radiation, why then did I eventually say a reluctant "yes" to both treatments? First, despite the ravages that I had read about, I hoped I could survive them; my will to live was strong.

Also, because doing it my way hadn't worked, I wasn't willing to continue alone any longer. As part of my decision-making process, I considered not only the cost of independent treatment vs a fully-funded cancer clinic protocol, but also the personal and relationship costs. In the end, I chose to allow my naturopath and the oncologists to chart my course.

Did I make the right decision? I don't know. But I know I did the best I could with the information I had. Plus, I'm still standing 13 years later. Although I have daily reminders in the form of a permanent colostomy bag, I'm enjoying my life with no cancer in sight.

Will what you pick work for you? I don't know that either. No one does. But if you base your decisions on your research and your feelings about what's right for you and your situation, you have as much chance of success as anyone.

Before this chapter ends, I want to say a bit more about "curing" cancer. One definition of the word "cure": *to make an illness or a medical condition go away*. Billions of dollars have been raised and spent on efforts to find "the cure". Let's face it. The war on cancer has been no more successful than the war on drugs.

I personally believe that we will never find "the cure" for cancer. Just as there will never be one truth in the world that works for all, there will never be **one** cure for cancer. Why? Because of the uniqueness in the way each of us is wired physically. Two people with the same type of cancer can respond differently to the same treatment and experience different results. When you factor in the mental, emotional, and spiritual aspects of every individual, the way through is much more complex.

What if we shift the focus to "healing" instead? To heal: "*to make someone who is ill become healthy again*." An individualized healing approach was the route that worked for me. In much of the rest of this book, we'll focuses on the roots of this eating-away disease called cancer.

Chapter 3
You & Your Healing Team

"Cancer cannot cripple love, it cannot shatter hope, it cannot conquer the Spirit." **Unknown**

Professionals

Regardless of your chosen treatment, it is essential to surround yourself with a team of practitioners that you respect, trust, and have faith in, because you will be seeing them on a regular basis. For example, if you have difficulty connecting with or trusting the first oncologist you visit, then request someone else. That is your right and your responsibility.

Supporters

Cancer is not just happening to you – you may be the one with the diagnosis, but your family and friends are on this journey with you. This is a rough journey to take alone. If you have no family close by, pick trusted friends with positive attitudes who will listen and help when needed.

One of the lessons I learned from cancer was the importance of receiving – of not being ashamed to ask for and accept help. Resist the urge to isolate or to maintain a fierce independence. I was humbled and astounded by the number of people who never hesitated to offer their services.

For your first oncology appointment, arrange for a driver/scribe to accompany you. Prepare your questions ahead of time. The job of your scribe involves taking notes and making sure all the questions are answered to your satisfaction. Trust me, the experience itself is too fresh and overwhelming to manage on your own. That focused recorder is there so you can concentrate on being present at your appointment. Also, having a driver will see you safely home.

I was asked by a friend with a breast cancer diagnosis to accompany her to her first appointment. She was well-prepared with her list of questions. I had my pen ready when the oncologist entered the room. After the briefest of introductions, the doctor began drawing diagrams on the board and describing what would happen next. Some of my friend's questions were brushed aside with a mumbled, "Oh, they'll tell you that in orientation."

It was obvious that this young woman was in a hurry to leave the room. She escaped as quickly as she could. When I noticed that not all the questions were answered, we had the nurse call the doctor back. Her "bedside" manner was not helpful. As a result, my friend requested a different oncologist – someone she felt had her best interests at heart and was willing to fully support her.

Some of your team will provide great emotional support; others will cook, drive, or clean your house. Who in your circle loves to make everyone laugh? Enlist their help with a "joke of the day" or something to raise your spirits.

This is the time to step away from toxic situations or relationships in your life – even if temporarily. You know who and what they are. Say no to the energy vampires – you will need every ounce of your energy! It's also important to keep in mind that you are not your cancer, even though it is in your body. Who you are is way more than any disease.

This Cancer Journey with Your Loved Ones

Several years after I healed from cancer, my sister got a nasty Stage 4 diagnosis of a rare and aggressive cancer for which there was no designated treatment that would work. Instantly I was thrust into the role of terrified supporter.

Because we were separated by distance (1800 miles), I encouraged her as best I could from afar. During the last eight months of her life, I visited twice – once to help with our parents while she was in hospital and then during the last two weeks of her life.

Helplessness is one of the most common feelings for supporters and caregivers. We don't know what to do, but we want to do *something* – anything to protect, shield, fix, comfort, support – in my case, because I'd successfully overcome my cancer, I was sure she'd turn to me for my knowledge and my experience.

But my sister was as fiercely independent as I had been. Not only was she deep in denial for the first year, but she was also determined to go through her cancer in her own way. My job was to provide loving support regardless of whether or not I agreed with her choices.

Each of us in the family helped in different ways. It was brutally hard to watch her suffering. None of us wanted to give up hope for a longer life for her, but at the end, all we wanted was for her to be at peace.

A cancer call is a prime opportunity to assess your relationships with loved ones. Maybe there are fences to mend. Maybe it's a time to re-connect or share what's on your mind and in your heart. "Nothing heartfelt left unsaid" became my mantra. Whether we have weeks or years more to live, what is the legacy of loving you want to leave behind?

As your loved ones walk this path with you, there will be times when it's all too much. Everyone will need a break, a change of pace, a change of scenery.

Spouses: While spouses usually have the largest role to play, it's unrealistic for them to handle everything all the time. In addition to assuming a caregiver role, they will have their own fears and challenges to deal with. Your spouse, most of all, will need someone to talk to about what they're dealing with.

You are **not** the best person to do this. You need all your strength and energy for you. I know I wanted my partner to be able to unburden without concern for my hurt feelings or damage to the relationship.

Encourage spouses to seek support from an outside source or ask other friends or relatives to help in this way. Your cancer center may have a psychologist or a group available for caregiver support that they can access. Remember that while he or she may be your biggest supporter, this cancer is happening to them, too.

Children: My son was 27 when I was diagnosed. When I was hospitalized, he'd stop by on his way home from work. He confessed to a friend of mine that he didn't know what to say to me – my friend assured him that it was his presence that was most comforting to me. I was glad that he had a spouse to share his thoughts with. I remember him running errands for me and making homemade soup.

I can only imagine a parent's concerns when young children are part of this journey. For a first-hand accounting, I recommend ***Run On, Amy*** a memoir by Phil & Amy Alain. They had two young children when Amy was diagnosed with inoperable lung cancer. Their book is filled with anecdotes of how each parent supported their kids through the stages of Amy's cancer.

Grown children with parents who have cancer can struggle mightily against the thought and fear of losing their loved ones. This is a time for courageous conversations where you can be frank about your needs, desires, and expectations.

While they may push for treatments to prolong your life, you may not want to be so sick that it destroys your quality of life and precious moments with children and grandchildren. Please muster up the courage to have a heartfelt conversation with your loved ones.

Friends: So many friends stepped up to help me. That didn't mean that their own life struggles disappeared while helping me or visiting me. One friend stopped herself mid-stream while sharing a tale of woe, "Oh, goodness. What I'm going through is so small compared to your problem." I encouraged her to keep talking.

We had always been each other's sounding board. Just because I was sick didn't mean she had to stop talking about what was important to her. Sharing her troubles took my attention away from my own – a welcome respite. I most wanted my friends to behave around me the way they always had.

If your friends know each other, encourage them to stay connected for their own moral support.

Siblings: It took a cancer diagnosis for me to understand how much my sister and brothers loved me. Although none of us lived in the same city, I knew they were there for me, just as we were there for my sister during her struggle with cancer. Because of all we've been through together, we are closer now than ever before.

Parents: A parent's worst nightmare is the thought of losing a child. A cancer diagnosis hits hard. One of the biggest challenges for parents is to resist interfering in the decisions of their grown children despite their fears.

Everyone has an opinion about a course of treatment – that doesn't mean it's appropriate to share unless asked. Scared though my dad was about my initial choices, he respected my decisions and offered only loving support.

Note: Because I've had no experience with young children who go through cancer and the anguish those parents experience, I've limited my thoughts to adults with cancer.

Chapter 4
The Process of Treatment

"Cancer is a marathon – you can't look at the finish line. You take it moment by moment, sometimes breath by breath, other times step by step." Sarah Betz Bulciere – caringbridge.org

Once Your Treatment Starts

Just as drug companies list potential side effects on pill bottles, you will get a list of possible reactions to your treatment. You may or may not lose your hair. Nausea may be minimal or terrible. Fatigue may be a constant companion.

The more you are aware of what could be ahead, the more prepared you can be to manage the aftereffects. Gather your key supporters ahead of time to share what you've learned about what's ahead and create a plan of action to manage your care.

My oncologist was very insistent about me taking my temperature regularly while on chemo. If it rose beyond a certain range, I was to head to Emergency immediately – there was even a special card to show the hospital staff. Do not ignore this instruction!

Toward the end of my chemo treatments, a raging infection spread throughout my body. When my temperature spiked one night, my spouse bundled me into the car and drove to the nearest hospital. Had I not gone to hospital then, you wouldn't be reading this book.

While it may not feel that way, your body is engaged in a mighty fight – the fight for survival. Cancer cells are particularly formidable and voracious, especially when they cluster. Like Pac Man, they gobble up every bit of energy available in order to mass produce.

Sugar is their fuel of choice, so I was advised to ditch the sugar in my diet. Since cancer cells don't use protein for energy, my doctor advised me to eat or drink as much protein as possible. Check with your doctor regarding protein recommendations and other dietary suggestions for your type of cancer.

Of course, eating enough and eating well is easier said than done when you have no appetite and feel like crap. A friend gave me a high-speed blender so I could drink my vegetables and protein and bump up my nutrition level.

We lose muscle mass when cancer strikes, so mild and consistent exercise like walking is important. When you feel awful, it's hard to get out of bed or off the chair, so you might need some motivation.

In advance of this fatigue, ask for help from one of your support team to walk with you. They are then available to go get the car if you can't make it back! While it's important to honor the new limitations of your body, it's also vital that you keep moving.

Pain medication may become your best friend. My oncologist (bless him) did not believe in me being in pain, so he made sure that I was pain-free. Although not normally a pill popper, in this case, I was most appreciative.

When Treatment is Complete

The end of my radiation treatments coincided with my release from hospital. I went home in a shell of a body that was barely functioning. Two flights of stairs greeted me.

No more meals delivered to my room, no cheerful and accommodating nurses to look after me, no more hospital routine or bustle – just deafening silence. I couldn't climb more than three stairs before sitting down. Making a meal took tremendous effort.

One of my hurdles was weaning myself off the potent pain killers. Morphine/Dilaudid side effects are nasty, and I had most of them. My oncologist warned me against going "cold turkey" and told me how to reduce the dosage gradually and safely. Withdrawal took an ugly six weeks, but I got through it. (Now I have a much better understanding of how people get hooked on drugs.)

Although I had a great many people willing to help, I had no plan for support once I went home. Bless those in my life who came forward unbidden and asked what I needed. If you have a plan, this is the time to activate your home support system.

- Who will drop off meals or shop for groceries?
- Who can drive you to your next appointment?
- Who would be a welcome visitor?
- Do you qualify for home care visits?

The NED Waiting Time

In my community, there is a big gap in psychological support from our medical service once treatment is finished. You are given a date for your next scan/appointment. In the meantime, you're on your own.

Patients wait with dread for that first test or CT scan to assess the effectiveness of treatment. I certainly did. I was scheduled every two months. As each appointment date loomed, I'd seize up with fear until the doctor reported "no evidence of disease" NED.

To me, it's as if fear is the bigger enemy here – not cancer.

No one told me how to deal with the time of uncertainty between test results. It felt as if my life was hanging in the balance with everything on hold. Lurking in the back of my mind was the dread I felt at the idea of cancer returning.

Dr. Kenford Nedd's book, *Power over Stress* talks about the parasympathetic nervous system in the body and its vital role in healing. This system shuts down when we're in fight, flight or freeze mode. Our storehouse of immune fighters depletes after three days. Plus, fear and prolonged stress impair the system's ability to replace those immune fighters. Hmm – no wonder our bodies struggle to heal!

These days, there are tools at our disposal to soothe the fear:

- Hypnotherapy
- EFT (Emotional Freedom Technique – Tapping)
- Havening
- Talk Therapy
- Tai Chi
- Qi Gong
- Yoga/Chair Yoga

Our minds and our emotions need healthy diversions between the routine appointments so that our fears don't take over. Support groups, painting lessons, journaling – check out what fits for you.

On YouTube, there are channels and videos about the above modalities. You can explore and experience many for free. If your medical plan covers the cost of paid professionals, it's worth the investment of time.

It's natural to want to be certain that the cancer, once gone, will never come back. But just as we don't know what day we will die; we won't know if cancer will come calling again. In my case, six months after radiation and chemo, the cancer came back in the same spot. As I mentioned, my only chance to remove the new spot was radical surgery. More fears and more healing to contend with!

In our "instant everything" society, we're not prepared to devote the time it takes to properly heal. It was six months after surgery before I started to regain weight – a vital body sign of returning to full health. It took even longer to recover muscle mass and stamina.

Eager to be a productive (money-generating) person again, I took on a full-time job four months after surgery – much too soon as it turned out. It took another year for full physical healing. Even though the doctors told me I was doing so much better than their other patients with the same cancer as me, my body felt very fragile during that time.

Addressing & Healing the Changes to Your Sexual Identity

Hesitant though I was to write about a subject that's rarely discussed among healthy individuals, never mind when it relates to healing from cancer, I was encouraged by two friends – both professionals in the medical field - to tackle the sensitive topic of loving and sexual functioning in the aftermath of resulting physical limitations.

At some point in your healing, you and a present or potential partner will be faced with the reality/possibility of intimate love after cancer.

Cancer and its treatment can alter us physically. In my case, at age 62, I was left with a radically shortened vagina plus the addition of an external rectum (called a stoma) protruding from my lower abdomen. Not only was I no longer capable of intimacy in the way of my youth, but my body also sported a permanent colostomy bag.

Accepting the physical reality of my condition took some time. Whenever I visited the bathroom or got undressed, I was reminded of my re-engineering. Emotionally, I had to work through the initial disgust I felt every time I saw this bag hanging beside my navel. I could clearly see that I had my poop in a group, and I wasn't happy about it!

Eventually, I came to some peace and acceptance about how I looked - even to the point of showering my naked body, bag and all in the presence of other women after swim class. I have had to work through any embarrassment I felt when disposing of my bags of human droppings at friends' homes.

From a romantic perspective, I felt like damaged goods – who would want me now?

Many women who have had mastectomies face similar emotional turmoil when they look in the mirror and see disfigurement where a beautiful breast once was.

Some women are fortunate enough to have strong partners whose love transcends what happened to their mates. Others endure the loss of relationships because of the surgery.

One of the challenges for women is believing their partners when told that they are still beautiful regardless of how their bodies have changed. If this is your challenge, please – believe your loved one – they are right! Our biggest enemy in this particular battle is ourselves.

I suspect that men with prostate or testicular cancer question their manhood and consequent lovability as well. Chemo cocktails can impair or cause the loss of sexual functioning. Skin can become either ultra-sensitive to the touch or have no feeling at all.

How do we navigate the murky waters of this vital and very sensitive arena? My initial attempt to research this topic did not meet with much success. Medical doctors receive roughly 10 hours of training about sexuality in general, never mind any training that would help their patients deal with sexual dysfunction.

Most of the books on store shelves have nothing to offer patients either. One good question for your oncologist is, "Who can help me regarding my sexuality questions in relation to cancer?"

When we reach a new intimacy crossroad, there are some choices. One choice has us abandoning sexual partnering and intimate connection altogether.

If we genuinely feel that we're ready to retire our sexual identity, there is absolutely nothing wrong with that choice. Many who make this conscious decision channel their attention and energy to other pursuits.

Another choice is that of self-love and love of our partner that leads to open, honest and vulnerable communication. For helpful advice about how to get started, I recommend you search for Joan Price on YouTube. She is a sexual specialist who works with adults over 60 who desire to commune sexually but are experiencing challenges they've never had before. Her videos and articles are down-to-earth and provide hope and encouragement.

In one of her recent posts, she recommended a book by Tess Deveze called, *A Better Normal – Your Guide to Rediscovering Intimacy After Cancer.* Tess is a breast cancer survivor and a physiotherapist whose specialty is sexual functioning for those with a variety of disabilities. She, too, counsels about the importance of communication to solve intimacy challenges.

I wonder how many singles and couples are suffering in silence and resigning themselves to a life without any kind of touch, be it sexual or comforting simply because no one knows how to talk about it.

Plus, our western society is so performance-based that whatever is outside the "norm" of sexual engagement is often labelled as not good enough. When really, love is love. If you feel adored and cherished by another person, even if that love is not expressed in a traditional way, is it any less loving or desirable?

Fear of either resuming intimacies with a current partner or starting a new relationship is a big obstacle because of how vulnerable everyone is in this arena. In an insane effort to protect us, fear encourages silence or distance and ignores how alone we feel. It would have us shy away from intimacy and settle for less than what we deserve.

Your partner is integral for support, but only you can do the work of accepting and loving the new you. Likely you will both work through the stages of grief as you come to terms with your – as Tess puts it "better normal".

I have always loved the definition of intimacy that goes: "into me see". That is really what happens when you allow or invite another to experience you at your most vulnerable.

Strange as it may seem, the more vulnerable you are willing to be, the stronger you and your relationship will become, both with yourself and with those closest to you. It's risky, but anytime I've allowed myself to be vulnerable in an intimate conversation, the other person and I got closer, not further apart.

Communicating your thoughts and worries to your loved one is the antidote to this fear. The light of heartfelt conversation will dispel the darkness of any fears. Many of our fears – *he/she will find me repulsive or unlovable now; I'll be rejected or see pity on their face; we won't be able to get past this* – those fears plus any others you can imagine will often dissipate as a result of some frank sharing. But you won't know that unless you talk it out. It will take courage, but then, you've already faced down cancer, so you have all the courage you need.

There are so many benefits to mind, body, and spirit as a result of deeply loving and being loved by another person. Our sexuality and sensuality are vital parts of our spiritual essence. We are sexual beings – it's important to honor our sexuality and sensuality, regardless of limitations.

When You aren't the Cancer Sufferer

What if you're the partner of someone whose body has been ravaged by disease or treatment? Damaged muscles need time to heal. Exhaustion requires recovery time. Libido seems to disappear or at least take a long vacation. Skin can be ultra-sensitive to touch. Pain may still be present. Those are just some of the physical realities he/she faces. I've already listed many of the emotional/mental barriers.

Cancer didn't just happen to your partner. It also affects you and it affects your relationship. Your needs and desires are as important as your loved one's needs. You, too, will grieve the loss of what you had before. Any limiting beliefs and fears of yours will rise to be dealt with.

Your role as lover and supporter will require much patience, understanding and honesty laced with a great deal of kindness and compassion. This is not a time to pull away or suffer in silence.

It will take time and effort from each of you to build a new life. Think about and then share what's most important to you now. Don't be shy about getting the help you need from professionals.

I know of couples who have done this work. It paid off handsomely in the form of an even deeper intimacy.

SUE PAULSON

The Face of Rage©

I could not see the face of rage

until cancer came knocking.

This rage had a magnificent beauty.

Fiery passion fueled by dark

and terror-driven thoughts.

Unleashed over the heads of

the unsuspecting

unsuspected even by the one afflicted with rage.

Bitter tears flowed

at the blow that Fate had dealt.

Why me? Why me?

What had I done that was so bad?

Then I looked, really looked at this face of rage.

Hurt lines filled with sorrow, abuse,

broken promises, betrayal, bitterness, and fear.

Fear of not being good enough -

never measuring up,

fear of never being seen or loved,

of being left out, shut out, ignored.

Fear of dying without ever having lived my heart's desire,

without ever having loved with ecstatic bliss.

Who knew that this rage was in me?

Will this ball of rage with its many faces consume me?

THE HEALING CALL OF CANCER

Choke me so I can't speak my Truth?

It's a fierce power, but not, I hope

more powerful than Love.

What if I allow rage

to rest in the palm of my hand,

stroke its surface with love and tenderness,

shine the light of Peace?

Noticed at last,

Will it start to soften and yield?

If I send it hope and understanding,

will it sigh with relief at being heard?

If I hold it close to my heart,

will it feel that soothing beat

and transmute itself to Joy?

Chapter 5
Exploring Thoughts & Feelings

"Don't move the way fear makes you move." Rumi

The mind is a curious thing. It is filled with our thoughts, feelings, emotions, and experiences. Larger than any computer database, it processes reams of information. To fuel and support our healing, we need the power of our minds – both our thoughts and our feelings to be our best friends.

Let's tackle feelings first. A variety of feelings are triggered by cancer – fear being the most primal of them. A deluge of negative thoughts and feelings that can happen at every stage of the cancer journey can swamp your boat if you allow it.

Hope vs Fear

My Grammy Ed had a saying for just about everything. One of her strongest beliefs was "Where there is life, there is hope." Amid my darkest fears, I clung to her belief as my life preserver.

To bolster my hope after diagnosis, I searched for information about people who had recovered from cancer. I read every story I could get my hands on about those who experienced miraculous healing and those who had been cancer-free for many years despite the odds stacked against them. It helped to ease my fear and build my determination to eliminate the cancer and to heal. Hope is one of the key antidotes to the terror you may be experiencing.

I come from a long line of "Where there's a will, there's a way" pioneers. While I did not know how to navigate through my adversity, this mantra kept the door open for solutions and possibilities, even though I couldn't immediately see them.

Thoughts

I once heard Daniel Goleman quote on Oprah's Super Soul Sunday: "No one knows enough to be pessimistic." He explained that we never know what good things might be around the corner, so our pessimism is always premature.

While there is no doubt that we have no way of knowing whether doom or joy is just around the corner, how does it serve us to continually dwell on doom and gloom thoughts? That choice then breeds even more doom and gloom that results in a downward spiral of misery.

While I was fighting for my life, I quit watching the news. You can see enough "Ain't it awful" stories on the nightly news to fill three lifetimes.

If there's any truth to the notion that "thoughts are things", then what are we creating with our thoughts? When we feel fear, thoughts of negativity, worry and anxiety, if we allow them, spread faster than quack grass with relentless roots that choke whatever is in its path.

We have had ample opportunities to become acquainted with our fear in other situations. Perhaps part of the healing that cancer brings is the opportunity to draw on our inner courage and stare down that fear or even befriend it.

With cancer, I certainly didn't know the way out initially, but I believed there was a way. That belief triggered another antidote: **knowledge**. We fear the unknown. Uncertainty dogs us. We hear a thump downstairs in the middle of the night. Our hearts pound until we investigate – only to find that the cat knocked something off the counter. We laugh with relief!

Most of what I knew about cancer was fear-driven media hype which suggested that cancer was a death sentence. Not true! Statistics showed that deaths from most kinds of cancer have been steadily declining since 1986. The more evidence I found regarding survivors, the stronger my hope became.

Out of the hope grew my faith – faith that I, too, could survive; faith that there was a way; faith that I would eventually find the gifts that this journey had to offer. I leaned heavily on other people's faith – especially when my own faltered.

In the twists and turns of this path, it's normal to stumble and fall. We need others to extend their hands. I had prayer warriors in churches I'd never been to, energy workers who surrounded me with healing vibrations, and family who held my hand and dropped off meals. All were important. I learned to welcome all of it.

Suffering in Silence

Suffering in silence was the way I thought I had to be when I got cancer. As a highly sensitive person, I felt the fear from family and friends when I told them of my diagnosis. Some people I told visibly shrank from me – as if they could catch cancer just by hearing me say the word!

Years later, after reading my book, *Magnificent Misery"* - a memoir of my cancer journey - loved ones said, "We had no idea that it was that bad for you." Of course, they had no idea – because I never told them. When I cried, I usually cried alone.

Looking back, I question my decision to suffer so much in silence. Obviously, if I had known differently, I might have done it differently, but I didn't, so it's futile to judge the way I handled it. But for you, my reader, I urge you to question your motives about being too silent. When you most need help, support, and protection, does it really serve all concerned for you to don the stoic mask or appear all happy and chirpy, no matter what? Put your pride in your pocket enough to be authentic and vulnerable – at least with those you trust the most.

Our loved ones can learn much from our suffering. Because of guilt and shame and in a misguided attempt to protect those around me, I may have robbed them of their own gifts from my experience.

Amy Alain, a lung cancer patient and co-author of the book, *Run On, Amy* always shared the truth with her young children of what was happening to her, right up to her dying day. Her kids proved to be stronger than she or her husband could have imagined.

There are such a myriad of negative emotions and thoughts to deal with in the early days. It can feel as if you're all alone in an ocean of uncertainty, with waves of fear, anger, and helplessness washing over you. I know I kept thinking that no one could understand what I was going through because they didn't have cancer.

While that may be partly true, every human being has faced some brand of adversity. Each has experienced pain, loss, trauma, and tragedy. That's the human condition. Because of their own experiences, people can relate. The ones who want to support you need to understand what you're going through. Yes, it's raw and real, but it's also authentic. Trust your supporters and acknowledge their strength.

I remember feeling guilty and ashamed that I had cancer. My guilt hung heavy, as if I had somehow betrayed my family by succumbing to something that I couldn't control. I felt like a burden when asking for help. I had always been the strong one – supporting but rarely needing or asking for support. In fact, I had always felt a certain pride in that strength, that I wouldn't have to be beholden to anyone.

Now I see that cancer was my opportunity to stop – just stop everything so I could focus on what was important in life. Who mattered, what mattered? Though embarrassed to ask for help, I asked anyway. Much to my surprise, my loved ones pitched in – with rides, with encouragement, with healing treatments, with research, with hugs and prayers. Their vigilance propped me up in my weakest, most hopeless moments.

Because I opened to receive, they were able to give. Though I judged myself, "What's wrong with me that I got cancer?", no one else did. They said, "How can I help? What do you need?"

Cancer is no different from any other adversity in that it brings us face to face with our mortality and gives us an opportunity to re-evaluate our lives and lifestyle. A classic example of that is my friend, Cal, a skilled herbalist and kinesiologist who treated my son in the mid 1980's. He shared his story when we first met.

He had been diagnosed with liver cancer in 1979. No treatment was available, so he was told to quit his high-stress job and get his affairs in order because he didn't have long. Determined to defy that diagnosis, he found a kinesiology institute in the States where they muscle-tested his system and filled him with appropriate herbs for healing.

It was a long road of focused attention on recovery. He became fascinated by the whole process, started learning what to do to help others, and eventually became a skilled practitioner. We met in 1987 when I was desperate for help for my son. From a death sentence to new life, Cal's not the only one who has healed from cancer and found a mighty purpose.

Let me repeat – if it's not your time to go, cancer won't kill you. However, when it is your time to go, cancer may very well be your ticket home. How you live in the meantime is up to you.

You may or may not have heard of Terry Fox, my favorite Canadian hero. That brave young man showed the world that meaning can arise from suffering. At the tender age of 18, he'd lost a leg to cancer. Even with the loss of one leg, he was determined to shine a light that would become a beacon of hope for other kids with cancer. He began an arduous run across Canada to raise awareness and funds for cancer.

Long after he was gone, the world remembered – they still remember every fall during the multitude of Terry Fox Marathons of Hope throughout North America.

He taught us much more than what it's like to have cancer. He taught us that it's not only possible, but desirable to find your own meaning and purpose in the face of the disease, regardless of how many days you have left on planet Earth.

Emotions

What if cancer is really our negative emotions personified?

If I am feeling dis-ease or uneasy about something – it's a vague feeling – it could be fear, frustration, anger, hurt etc. When I allow that out – maybe express it and then seek the root of it for resolution, then my body – the amazing barometer that it is – senses the danger is over and moves from high alert back to a sense of homeostasis or equilibrium.

When we don't deal with any dis-ease such as unresolved anger, resentments, unhappiness, bitterness and/or fears, they build up over time, causing the body to deal with chronic rather than temporary stress.

This compromises the body's ability to maintain itself at an optimal level. Immune fighters are overwhelmed and/or depleted, leaving the body with a limited capacity to eliminate damaged or rogue cells. At that point, there are places in the body that become fertile ground for the proliferation of disease – any kind of disease.

Why are statisticians now predicting that 1 in 2 will face cancer in their lifetime? I don't know, but what if one reason is because a cancer diagnosis scares the living daylights out of us – nothing else has been strong enough to grab our attention. This 2 X 4 called cancer hits us right between the eyes. "Wake Up!" it seems to say.

Now that our previously ignored fears have escalated into sheer terror – what happens next? It's only natural that our defense mechanisms are screaming to kick it – the ego pushes us to fight, flee, or freeze. It's interesting that all those defense strategies will only work temporarily.

Oh, we can label cancer our enemy and go to war with all the lethal medical weapons at our disposal – I tried them all – but all that deals with is the consequence, the result of a long journey living in a self-created hell.

THE HEALING CALL OF CANCER

Here's the interesting thing. If they don't kill us, current treatment protocols can buy us precious time to sort ourselves out, to get to the root cause(s) instead of just dealing with the symptom called cancer.

Personally, I believe that cancer is one sign that says we are not living the joyous life we were intended to live. I know I wasn't. Cancer was the pause button I needed to examine what was and wasn't working.

Sadly, many cancer sufferers weather the invasive treatments and the aftermath of debilitation without ever understanding that cancer has provided an opportunity for a do-over. My life had been tough for many years – some of it because of circumstances that felt beyond my control. The rest of it was because of self-imposed limitations and fears.

Compared to many whose lives were much worse, my life didn't look or feel that bad, but it was bad for me. My body knew this – it kept sending signals that I ignored until the cancer came.

I was fortunate that a near-death experience four years prior to cancer opened my eyes to the ecstasy of life that was possible and the realization that my life did not match that level of bliss. The potential for joy and thrival was there, but I had been so stuck in survival that I couldn't find it in me to move toward what my soul most craved.

Cancer was akin to the match that lit my rocket fuel. Though I didn't know it at the time, I was jet-propelled toward my own healing.

From knowledge and experience gained over the years about the mind-body-soul connection, I knew that a return to full health wasn't just about killing cancer cells. Intuitively, I knew the most important work would begin after surgery. Serendipitously, the day before surgery, I found a healing lifeline.

Chapter 6
Exploring & Changing Our Minds

"You have to be willing to give up the life you planned, and instead, greet the life that is waiting for you." Joseph Campbell

As soon as I could sit comfortably after surgery, I started sessions with Dr. Francisco Valenzuela, a hypnotherapist who specialized in working with oncology clients. A friend had sent me the link to his website.

With his help, I turned inward to my thoughts and feelings. We rooted out old, mistaken beliefs (I'm not worthy, I don't deserve etc.) and examined the feelings that were right beside them.

Lifelong patterns coalesced to form my path to cancer. Schooled and conditioned very young to serve others first and foremost, I had given too much, felt unworthy, hung out in self-denial, and asked for too little.

I saw everyone else's potential but was blind to my own. While others feasted at the banquet, I, with a smug kind of self-righteousness and martyrdom, settled for the crumbs under the table.

Rage and lifelong resentments had gradually fueled those rogue cells and made them as tough as steel plates. I have come to believe that when you feel sick at your heart and soul level, the physical manifestation of something nasty can certainly follow.

Once I identified the beliefs and thoughts that had been slowly killing me, I began the process of inner transformation and healing. I journaled, I read, I meditated, and I dreamed about my heart's desire for my life.

It took about two years of self-reflection to build in my mind my idea of heaven on earth. I expect it will take the rest of this lifetime to create it.

Because it's been possible for me, I know it's possible for you as well. Now that you've had that whack on the side of your head, what will you do next? If you have no clue – read on. What has worked for me just might work for you, or perhaps one of my ideas will lead you to your own great idea!

Joyous Life

"I don't know how to live a joyous life," said my elderly aunt recently. I was sad for her, and I'm sad for anyone who struggles and stresses and can't seem to find any joy in life. I too, have had those moments.

In the face of all the joy and goodness in the world, why do we find ourselves wallowing in what's wrong? Instead of running toward the light, we flee from one darkness to another. We lead lives filled mostly with trauma and drama.

The cycle of pain can be so intense that some succumb to a variety of addictions. For a time, we might think we feel better, but our bodies won't be tricked. Bless our bodies – they keep working miraculously - until they don't. When they send us the biggest message we've ever received, it's time to pay attention.

The story of Pollyanna clearly demonstrated the route to a joyous life. I was about 10 when I saw the movie. Maybe you've even read the book by Eleanor H. Porter. Briefly, the story is about a sunny, exuberant 10-year-old girl who had been tragically orphaned and impoverished and was sent to live with a wealthy aunt who was not only strict, but very bitter about life.

Before he died, Pollyanna's father - a preacher - had taught her "the glad game". Whenever she was sad or feeling bad about some situation, he showed her how to look for something to be glad about. It was a simple, yet very effective recipe for living joyously.

Even though she had a tough time adjusting and was in trouble frequently due to her "odd" ideas, it never stopped her from looking for the good in life and in people, and guess what? She found it!

Despite more adversity and trauma that dogged her footsteps, she clung to her "glad game". Her outlook on life at such a young age seeded my own.

One secret to living a joyous life is to look for joy and smile when you find it. Joy is all around us, but it doesn't announce itself like a big brass band.

It's a whisper in the breeze, a delicate flower just coming into bloom, soft rain, or warm sun on your face. Even if you are experiencing great tragedy, trauma, or loss, you are still surrounded by joy. It never stops being there, though you may be too immersed in darkness to notice it.

"But, Sue," you say. "My life is a mess. There are so many things wrong, I can't even count them." Well, I may not have experienced exactly what you're going through, but I do understand because my life has been filled with lots of suffering, too.

As much as I might curse the Gods and wish it were otherwise, I'm not sure we came to planet Earth to have an easy time of it. Great contrast such as that between dark and light help us choose our direction in life. Out of the biggest adversity of my life came the greatest gifts.

Gratitude

Here's what I did to re-discover my joy. I started a list in my head and then in my journal of everything that I was grateful for in any given moment. Even if things were bleak, I always found something.

I can still bend over to put my socks on; there's enough cereal in the box for breakfast; my wonky battery in my car still works; the sun is shining; my kid made his bed without me nagging; I got an unexpected cheque in the mail.

When we're grateful for even the smallest thing, it chips away at our misery and starts to ease the pain. The more I do this little exercise, the more joyous I feel. The more joyous I feel, the more I think differently about my situation, so there's a turning away from the darkness I've been in. More often than not, little miracles occur, and things change for the better.

Success as an Inside Job

We're taught very young that results are what matter - that the success of a person is measured by the good deeds and accomplishments that society deems valuable.

Get a good education, get an even better job, make lots of money, marry the "right" person, buy a house, two cars, have the requisite 2.5 kids (how does that work?!) – well, you get the picture. If that spells success, then I don't qualify.

I never went to university, I've been divorced twice, never held down a "job" with one company for more than five years, lost two houses, went bankrupt twice and only had one child. Does that make me a loser in society's eyes or in the eyes of my family? Maybe.

But the important question to me is whether I am a success in my own heart and mind. Blanche, a very wise 103-year-old friend said, "You have to live your own life, no matter what anyone else says." That's what I've been doing – living my own life.

Because of all the experiences in my life, I'm happy – sometimes for no apparent reason. For me, success is an inside game.

What about for you?

- Do you determine your worth by what you know about you inside of you?
- Are you better today at loving and understanding than you were yesterday?
- Do you value yourself, your talents, skills, and experience?
- Do you believe yourself to be worthy of all good things?
- Are you following your passions and dreams?
- Are you happy with your choices?
- Do you see yourself as a victor of your own life rather than a victim of circumstances?
- Do you live your values?
- Are you in integrity with your own purpose and reason for being?
- Do you feel safe to show up as your raw, real, and authentic self?

Even though we will never know how far our light will shine outwardly, the first step is to let it shine from within.

Chapter 7
Thoughts Become Things

"We may not be responsible for the world that created our minds, but we can take responsibility for the mind with which we create our world."
Gabor Mate, Physician/Author

How we see ourselves and how we talk to and about ourselves will have an impact on cancer healing. Are we worthy? What do we deserve? How strong are we really in this fight for our lives?

There were two key learnings for me during my cancer journey. First, I learned that I was terrible at asking for or receiving help. After that first diagnosis, out of necessity I gradually opened myself to all kinds of support. Initially, I accepted with a feeling of shame until friends said, "Sue, you've been giving all your life. Now it's our turn to give to you." So, reluctantly, and begrudgingly, I received their help.

When my cancer came back after six months of being clear, I felt like such a failure that I didn't even want to tell my loved ones. Why not? Because I really believed that since I had failed, I was unworthy of people's precious time or support.

As I heard myself utter that thought to my partner, I was stunned to hear those words come out of my mouth. Unworthy – really? Obviously, I had more to learn. Cancer was proving to be a mighty teacher!

As an avid student of human nature and human behavior, I have always been fascinated by the studies about mind-body connections. For example, scientists know that even a fake smile sends a shot of endorphins – those feel-good hormones – into the body that helps it re-vitalize. On the other side, fear causes our hearts to pound and creates a stress response – dis-ease. If left to build, that dis-ease can grow into disease – cancer being one of them.

Dr. David R. Hawkins, in his work on the evolution of consciousness, created a chart that divides common feelings into two categories: life-enhancing and less than life-enhancing. The destructive emotions include anger, fear, guilt, and shame. The positive emotions include peace, joy, love, and acceptance.

Experiencing negative emotions in the moment is not the problem. It's when we hang onto them and continue to judge ourselves – then we can be in trouble. Personally, I had unknowingly carried deep shame and guilt from childhood. I had also nursed anger, bitterness, and resentment toward my parents and God. All of it was fertile ground for cancerous growth.

Reversing my thoughts, healing those old wounds, and shifting my emotions from negative to positive brought me out of my self-imposed suffering so I could fully heal. You, too, have the power to bring yourself out of your own darkness and into the light of healing.

In case you didn't know or have forgotten – you are a **magnificent** creation – worthy of everything you might ever desire. What will you choose to create next?

Changing States of Being

Greg Braden, in a recent interview stated quite clearly that we are in charge of our thoughts, our feelings, and our beliefs. If we're in charge, then that means we can change anything that is less than life-enhancing.

Picture yourself in the grocery store. Before you is a vast array of products ready for you to take home. Different labels and items are stacked throughout the aisles. When something captures your attention – maybe it's on your list – into the cart it goes.

But you don't own it yet. You could change your mind and put it back. You only own what's in your basket once you've paid your hard-earned cash.

Thoughts are like that. We're exposed to a myriad at any given moment – in fact bombarded with them. But none of them belong to us unless we take ownership. How do we do that? First, we judge the thought – good/bad, right/wrong etc. Then we attach an emotion to it. That gives it energy. (Emotion is energy in motion.) When a thought is combined with some emotion, it tends to stay at the front of our minds.

One example is how we think about ourselves. When I was a young teenager, I compared my body to those of friends and family and judged that I was overweight, which I then felt "bad" about. I had that thought, the resulting judgment created a negative feeling, and ultimately, I adopted the belief that I was somehow deficient because my body was not an "ideal size". (My mother was tall and thin – a model's figure, while I was short and curvy.)

In my late twenties, I found a picture of my 17-year-old self whom I had previously perceived to be short, fat, and dumpy. There I was – slim and pretty! I could hardly take in what I was seeing. My years-long belief about myself simply wasn't true. However, the pattern of belief and resulting body shame was set – a pattern I still struggle to change.

The strange thing is, there are many ideas that we change our minds about constantly and easily. It should naturally follow that we could simply change our minds about our self-perception when we are in error. Although it sounds simple, changing a lifetime of negative perceptions about yourself will take focus and effort.

Now is the time to be your own best friend – that friend who adores you, admires and respects you and believes that all your good qualities far outweigh any judgments you have about quirks and foibles. If you aren't that friend yet, maybe it's time.

The following are some exercises that helped me become my own best friend.

1. Get to Know You

Find a scribbler, or better yet, a nice journal. Your challenge is to list at least 100 things you like about yourself. Start by writing the numbers 1 -100 with room to write beside each number.

Starting at #1, write down a good point about yourself. Anything goes here – physical characteristics (long eyelashes, cute nose) personal attributes (honesty, kindness) life skills (cooking, driving) talents (music, sports) professional skills (keyboarding, communicating) – explore all categories and get very detailed!

There are two tricks to getting to the first 100. Be as specific as possible and ask for help when stuck. Maybe there are 20 physical characteristics you like – list them all. When you get stuck (I got stuck several times) ask someone you trust to help. Explain the exercise and then ask them to provide a good point – they always supply more than you think they will.

Note: If it would take you less than 5 minutes to list 100 things you **don't** like about yourself, then this exercise is extra important for you!

1. Acknowledge Your Achievements

Turn to a new section of your journal.

Now I want you to remember and write down the achievements you've had from the beginning of your life. (This will be a long list if you're over 21!) Did you learn to read, ride a bicycle, start a campfire, learn to play a musical instrument? When did you win your first level of a computer game, get your first girlfriend/boyfriend, score an A in one of your school subjects?

Many of our seemingly small victories build on each other – because you achieved this, you were able to achieve that. When we focus on and acknowledge the vast amounts of things we have learned to do, it builds our self-confidence and helps us trust our abilities to learn more.

For example, the applause I received for memorizing and reciting a poem at church when I was only 10 fueled a desire to be a speaker at the front of the room. Who knew then that speaking to audiences would become one of the most joyful ways I earn my living!

The more often you start your day focusing on the good that you are, the more powerful you will feel. It stops the downward spiral into bitterness and depression and fuels your hope, determination, and faith in yourself.

1. Play the Dreaming Game

It's your life – if you don't decide what's meaningful for you to fill your days, someone else will. (You may not like what they pick!)

The point is to dream – in an ideal world – your brand of heaven on earth - what would you like to be, have, and do that is not in your sphere right now? What have you stopped yourself from wanting, never mind doing? Refuse to let those "ya but's" take over. "Ya, but I don't have enough_____". There's an old saying, "Argue for your limitations, and they're yours." Haven't you limited yourself enough?

I confess – I've dreamed many times about what I would do if I won the lottery – something about renting a Lear jet and taking friends to Paris for lunch! Beyond that, I've also envisioned my heart's desire for my life – the work I love that will make the world better, places I want to visit, the people I want surrounding me.

Your ideal world could be a better lifestyle for you and your family, and/or it could include a vision for the change you want to make in the world. Earlier in this book, I mentioned a recent addition to my bookshelf, Run On, Amy by Phil & Amy Alain. This is a memoir about Amy's cancer and her subsequent vision for shining the light on the stigma of and lack of funding for lung cancer research. Through social media, she posted videos of her daily Lunges for Lungs.

While undergoing treatment, she also noticed the lack of accommodations for out-of-towners undergoing cancer therapy. Amy's House is the result of Phil Alain's desire to fulfill one of his wife's dying wishes. Amy was 39 when she passed, yet she lives on through the impact she made and continues to make in others' lives.

Whether you journal about or create a vision board for your heart's desires, mark your calendar to review them every three months. The fun part is checking off what has already been achieved! I am still astonished when I discover that so many of my dreams have not only come true but manifested more quickly than I might have imagined. They wouldn't have, though if I had never dreamed them in the first place.

Out of Judgment Toward Compassion

I recall judging myself even more harshly after the cancer diagnosis than ever before. It seemed like the ultimate punishment (for what I couldn't imagine) but I assumed I must have done something really bad – hadn't I? I'd eaten too much junk food, had not exercised enough – it served me right – it was all my fault – blah, blah, blah!

Not only was the judgment wrong, but it also served no good purpose. Blame and shame have no place on this healing journey. What we need most is loving compassion.

I doubt that most of us get up in the morning with the intention to screw up royally. When we can find it in our hearts to be o.k. with our mistakes and recognize that if we had known at the time how to do it better, we would have, then forgiveness is easier and the next natural step. There is a big difference between being "at fault" and being "the reason".

Because I exist and I have free will to make choices, I am the reason for all the results I have in my life, both what I like and what I don't like, what worked and what didn't. If a result is not to my liking, I can simply choose again. Life is all about experimenting.

But if we judge ourselves – It's all my fault, that was wrong, I'm bad – it triggers an endless loop of guilt and/or shame that prevents us from learning the routes to more productive outcomes. Let me point out here that feeling remorse for having behaved badly is healthy and much different from blame and shame.

I'm sure you've noticed that we're surrounded by blame and judgment. Many of the negative self-concepts we hang onto were seeded by parents and authority figures when we were too young to know the truth or had no ability to exert our power.

But once we see how harmful those judgments are, we get to choose what we will do moving forward. It's not only our right but our responsibility to let go of what is past and to chart a new course toward the magnificence we really are.

Selective Forgetting

Like jigsaw puzzle pieces, the big picture of each of our lives is an accumulation of every experience throughout our time here, whether we label it "good" or "bad". When we re-visit the great times, it's a happy trip down memory lane. The tough parts of the story though can continue to trigger pain and cause us to stay stuck if we don't work to either re-frame the experiences or let them go.

While everyone's trials and tribulations are different, pain is pain and wounded emotions happen to us all, regardless of the circumstances or the degree. If that pain is preventing you from moving forward, you will love the gifts that come from facing what's there and dealing with it.

Let me share a personal example to illustrate this. I have had three long-term relationships in my life - two formal marriages and one common-law relationship – a total of 36 years in coupledom. At the end of each of those relationships, I felt very keenly not only the loss of the good parts of being in an intimate relationship, but I felt guilt and shame for not being able to live happily ever after with any one of them.

There were also varying degrees of anger toward each partner for the role they had played in my perceived victimization. This is often the point where couples get stuck. I know people who still speak of their former partners with huge bitterness even 20 years after the divorce.

Personally, I don't see the point of terminating an unhealthy relationship only to stay mentally and emotionally attached! If that isn't hell on earth, I don't know what is. I'm grateful I was able to remain friends with former partners.

For a time, I felt justified in my anger and hurt. I wanted to blame them for the problems – but my Spirit kept reminding me of my own contribution to the break-up. A desire to understand and learn from what went wrong helped me to see my partners' points of view.

Eventually, I was able to forgive them and forgive myself. Ultimately, I came to understand that we had chosen each other in order to grow – there was really nothing to forgive.

The selective forgetting came later – what I mostly remember now about the relationships are the good times we had and how much I benefitted from each of those relationships. What a relief for me to lay down that bundle of suffering.

It sounds simple, doesn't it? Just let all that crap go and get on with your life cheerfully and joyfully. Well, it is simple, but sometimes our stories wind around us so tightly that we can't find the thread that would start the unraveling. While I have not found that level of letting go to be easy, it has been worth the price of time and effort.

To begin, you have two very powerful tools at your disposal. One tool is called **self-love**. You cannot be your own best friend if you don't love yourself. Think about it - when you love your pet turtle more than you love yourself, maybe it's time to take action.

Forgiveness is the other powerful tool. When we forgive someone, it's not that we condone or absolve that person of his/her actions or behavior, it's that we let go of or surrender the burden of the situation. We find a new understanding and compassion that helps us lighten our own load.

One excellent way to start resolving a painful past is through the exercises in Byron Katie's book, *Loving What Is*. Her simple exercises will take you on a journey that will bring realization and help you to move out of that suffering space that you feel trapped in. If you don't relate to her message, there's plenty of help online or at your local bookstore. Notice what calls to you.

Over the years, in my quest to reduce my pain and suffering and increase my joy in life, I have experienced many different methods and modalities. Sometimes I would rocket forward and other times I would stumble, fall, and start again. And that's okay. Life is messy. There are no manuals that avoid pitfalls, roadblocks, and detours.

The good news is that others like me have figured a few things out and are here to help, guide, and assist. If you remember nothing else, remember that you are not alone on this journey. Help is available - just reach out and ask for it.

Be prepared for your ego to prevent you from ditching those painful stories. It will try to tell you that you will disappear if you let go of those stories. Who will you be if you're not angry and miserable? Who would you be under all that you have ever suffered? It's You, Magnificent You!

Chapter 8
A Trip to Heaven

"Heaven lives forever in our heart. This is how we create Heaven on Earth – through our heart." Roxana Jones/roxanajones.com

Who You are as Spirit

At some point in your cancer journey, you may choose to explore facets of your spiritual nature. I have found this inward journey to be intensely rewarding, because it provided understanding and insight that was critical to my evolution.

What is this essence we call Spirit? From a cosmic perspective, it has been labelled God, Allah, Source, the Universe, the Other Side, The Great Beyond. Regardless of the label, to me, it's the macro to our human micro. On our human level, since we are a part of it all, I believe it's the highest, most knowing part of us that is connected to Universal Consciousness. My understanding is that all of us came from, are connected to, and will return to that Source – Eternal Life.

My youthful understanding of God was that we were separate. He was way up there, that white-bearded guy in the sky, and if I wanted his attention, I would have to be good, measure up – do things he deemed worthy enough in order to grant me a seat at the celestial banquet table.

Schooled in the Anglican faith, I was taught that I was a miserable sinner with a lengthy road to become worthy of God's regard. While I didn't feel like a sinner at 14, I did feel miserable. My relationship with God was tentative at best. I did my best to "measure up" but it never seemed enough.

My spiritual awakening came four years before cancer, in July 2007. I had a near death experience that shattered all my former beliefs about God and the Universe, and more particularly, my part in the Grand Scheme.

Emergency surgery sent me to the Other Side where that Soul part of me basked in a sea of unconditional love. Never had I experienced that level of love before! Along with the love was pure acceptance. Judgment did not exist. There was no book of reckoning to label us good or bad, as either saints or sinners. There was also no requirement to have lived a certain way in order to measure up, because there was nothing to measure up to. Each Soul was a shining and integral facet of the Universal Diamond – fully worthy because it existed.

As wrapped up in my feelings and beliefs as I was, it was difficult to grasp that Consciousness is neutral about our choices. Growth is the prime directive. Regardless of the direction of each Soul's choice, every result contributes to the Whole. Free will is without conditions.

Regardless of the human labels of saint and sinner, everyone has a seat at the celestial table as an equal. Just as snowflakes are unique and contribute to the snowbank, each human makes a unique and magnificent contribution to the universe. That's what I experienced, understood, and felt at a soul-deep level.

That time in "Heaven" was the full-blown ecstasy I had been searching for my whole life – pure bliss! So, you can imagine how tough it was after surgery to return to self-created misery. Even though re-entry was painful and certainly didn't feel like my choice (I felt as if I had been voted off Paradise Island!) I had the sneaking suspicion that it was all part of some divine plan.

Stripped of mistaken beliefs, I entered a period many would call the "Dark Night of the Soul". What was left if there was never any obligation to prove my worth? Had the ways I'd served for years been for no reason? With my previous foundation collapsed, what was the meaning and purpose of my life?

Though I functioned well enough on the surface, this internal struggle continued until cancer came calling in February of 2011. Looking back, I can't help but feel that my trip Home in 2007 was preparation for the epic battle to come. Fearful though I was about the cancer diagnosis, I no longer feared death. If cancer took me Home – I won. If I survived it – I won.

Will and Power

Your ability to heal is connected to your will and your belief in the power of your own spirit. Let's talk about power first. One definition: *a natural or special ability to do something – the ability to control events - unknown or magical forces that people believe can influence events in a good or evil way.* While everyone has plenty of personal power, you can only exert as much as you believe you have.

In my childhood and teens, I felt I had very little power over anything. After attending my first personal growth program in my 20s, I realized I had way more power than I had ever given myself credit for. I wasn't sure where this power came from, but I suspected it wasn't just from little ol' me.

Using that power to solve problems, find peace, and manifest what I wanted was heady stuff. It was so easy that it felt like cheating – as if I had discovered an advantage no one else had. What interfered with this newfound sense of power was an old belief that in order to achieve what I wanted, it would have to be at someone else's expense – my gain, their loss. Because I couldn't reconcile this power in light of my beliefs, I was afraid and used it sparingly.

Eventually I came to know that every person on the planet has this power. Whether they ever find it, believe it, or choose to use it (for good or evil) it's an inherent part of that person's own will.

Will relates to determination to do something – regardless of the level of difficulty. If you have a strong will to live, that serves you well in the face of cancer. When we put the two words together ***will power***, it sets our course in a specific direction. We fire up our energy to do what's necessary, despite how hard it might be.

In the early days of cancer, I remember not knowing which way to turn – which course of action would be the best for me. I also remember being determined: "I will find a way." "I will get through this." "I will get off this morphine." "I will find out what started this journey."

It took great fortitude in the face of plenty of pain and several setbacks. Despite my will and my knowledge of my own power, I was scared. What I knew scared me, and what I didn't know also scared me. There were times when it was only the determination of others that kept me going. Deep despair hit at different times. Endless pain coaxed me to give up and let go. There were moments when the idea of death seemed like a welcome relief.

Still, I soldiered on. I clung to every crumb of hope there was. I wore the prayer shawl I'd been given and mostly just endured whatever was in front of me.

Twenty months from my first diagnosis, I was cancer-free. The journey was not the way I had envisioned it. It was messy, it was brutally hard, and because of the recurrence, I lost precious body parts and had to be re-engineered through surgery. But the goal – to live through it – was achieved.

Since my recovery in 2012, I've looked at will and power and have come to know that both of those came to me from Spirit. I believe the Divine Intent was for me to live through cancer in order to fulfill my mission on earth – to complete what I'd come here to do. I did live through cancer, and now, through cancer, I'm learning how to live.

On Star Trek, they used to talk about the final frontier. Although they were referring to outer space. I believe our final frontier is our inner world - the heart of us, the root of us that is connected to Source.

Scientists are beginning to confirm that it is through our hearts that this contact is made. It's the place where we are face to face with our Essence, our Beingness where we discover and really know, perhaps for the first time, what magnificent creations we are.

So how then do we embrace this larger-than-life idea of ourselves? If we don't have a developed sense of our own worth, we need to replace old, disempowering beliefs with new empowering ones. In AA, they call it doing a fierce, moral inventory. Others call it the Dark Night of the Soul.

Regardless of the name, the work is the same. We dig deep in order to grow. Think of it as the garden of our Being. Fertile soil (our minds and hearts) can grow anything - including weeds that take over and choke the life out of every good thing we want.

Some of this unwanted stuff takes root when we're too young and vulnerable to stop it or even realize that it is not good for us. We do what we're told; we also believe most of what we're told to believe. Noxious weeds of self-doubt and low self-esteem can fill our gardens without us even realizing it.

When we start to contemplate, to question, to seek - that's when we get ready to till the soil and remove whatever doesn't belong in our patch of paradise. In Louise Hay's book, "Heal Your Body" she gives the underlying mental state that seeds the ground for cancer: *Deep hurt. Longstanding resentment. Deep secret or grief eating away at the self. Carrying hatreds. "What's the use?"*

When I read that passage in her book, I resonated strongly with all of it. Most of my deep hurts and resentments stemmed from early childhood. Those early seeds took root and resulted in my belief that I was not worthy - of love, of esteem, of health, of wealth - of any of the wondrously glorious flowers of life.

That belief led to the thought that cancer was my punishment - that I deserved all the pain and anguish of the disease and the treatment because of something I had either done or failed to do. Somehow it was all my fault.

Of course, none of those assumptions were true. Cancer was not a punishment nor was I to blame for having it. Instead, it was my wake-up call - my opportunity to walk the garden of my life to see what had taken root. Regardless of whether or not I had personally seeded those weeds, my new awareness clearly showed that I was responsible for ridding myself of noxious stuff.

Gabor Mate, M.D. in his book "The Myth of Normal" along with his colleague, Bessel A. Van Kolk – "The Body Keeps the Score" firmly point to research and case studies that confirm one of the key roots of dis-ease which leads to disease is **trauma,** especially early childhood trauma.

While I didn't have the benefit of Mate's or Van Kolk's knowledge during my cancer journey, my intuition helped me find the help I needed for full healing. Through multiple sessions, psycho-oncologist and hypnotherapist, Dr. Francisco Valenzuela showed me how previous childhood emotional traumas had seeded the ground for cancer to grow within me.

A great beginning for any cancer sufferer questing to heal would be to consider the questions "Do I love Me? How much? If the answer is no or not much, then chances are pretty good that you have some weeds strangling your belief in your own magnificence and worthiness.

Never doubt that you deserve all the love there is. Why? Because you exist - you are here! There is nothing to earn, nothing to do - it is your birthright.

If you find yourself ready to argue with the above paragraph, congratulations! Prove me wrong if you can. Better yet, prove me right! I know how much love I deserve. And I know how much love you deserve - all there is. The beauty of love is that there is an endless supply. It will never run out.

Once I began to accept and really feel my worthiness, the wonder of me and my life plus its glorious possibilities began to shine through. All of it is there for you, too - your personal version of Heaven on Earth.

Chapter 9
You -Creator of Your Own Reality

"I've been searching for ways to heal myself, and I've found that kindness is the best way."

Lady Gaga

Cancer as Teacher

Let's move along the healing path one step further. What if I told you that you (unconsciously, unknowingly and for your highest good) brought in your cancer – that you invited it in as your teacher?

It's a strange notion – right? Perhaps you feel a sense of indignation or anger at this very thought. I confess that when this idea first flitted through my head, I pushed it away as quickly as it came. I thought to myself, "Who would do such a terrible thing to themselves and those around them?"

My judging mindset felt that if I took full responsibility for this creation, then I must shoulder the blame. But what happens if we suspend judgment, remove blame, and simply become curious about this idea.

As powerful Beings, if you were the cause of your cancer and I was the cause of mine, then perhaps we can also heal it. What if there are countless gifts to come because of our experience with this adversity?

As I healed both physically and emotionally, I began to explore this idea more fully. Through work with my hypnotherapist, I learned that my emotional and mental state stemming from a marriage breakdown eight years earlier had set up fertile ground for cancer to grow. That made sense to me. Further digging revealed that even earlier patterns of negative and mistaken beliefs had prepared the soil for that cancer.

I could clearly see that the consequences of my previous state of being had led me to cancer. While I resonated with that from an emotional and mental perspective, I wondered about the spiritual component.

Thus, my deeper spiritual journey began. I had many questions about the nature of God and my place in the Universe. Why was I here? Did my purpose matter? Did I matter? This quest began in earnest about a year after my surgery. I found many of my answers in Neale Donald Walsch's book, "*Communion with God*".

As you can imagine, all this soul-searching churned up old beliefs and programs that were obstacles to my growth. One by one, I worked through them.

As I let go of what didn't serve me, I started to find more peace. I learned how to be happy. I found joy in the simplest things. I came to love myself in the most beautiful way. Even better, I started to open up to the possibility of a personal, loving relationship with the God of my understanding.

One of my past mentors likened this process to peeling the layers of an onion until you get to the nut of it. I must have the biggest onion known to man, because the layers still seem endless, no matter how many I peel! I confess that I am still peeling and still growing in 2023.

If it feels right to you, I encourage you to explore your spiritual nature. Cancer led me there. What I discovered has been one of my greatest gifts.

We're conditioned to fight – but is it right?

There have been many times in my life when I finally stopped fighting the inevitable. My cancer diagnosis was one of those. I fought the reality of the symptoms for years. When the news was delivered, I couldn't and wouldn't believe it, so for a while, I fought that. There was no denying the evidence though, so eventually I surrendered to the fact of having cancer in my body.

The old adage that I grew up with, "When the going gets tough, the tough get going" is one way of handling things. Adversity has always raised the hackles on the back of my neck and triggered my fighting instinct. Every ounce of my will became focused on overcoming or battling the obstacles in front of me.

Sometimes I would win, sometimes I would lose. Regardless, there was a price to pay for all that fighting. In retrospect, I see that many times the cost was intense and needless suffering.

I remember reading about the miraculous, spontaneous healing of cancer in Anita Moorjani's case. As her organs shut down and she was dying, she had her own trip to the Afterlife. Not her time to "die", she re-entered her body, which healed spontaneously over the next six months.

Because I knew that same power was available to me, it bothered me that my journey was so messy and so tough. I thought there was something wrong with me that I couldn't just "image" the cancer gone. I wanted to have my prayers for instant healing answered as others had.

I know now that each journey has its own path and purpose – all for the good of the sufferer. Much as I didn't like it, my higher purpose was better served by the healing path I chose.

Cancer has been my biggest battle to date. But it wasn't a battle with cancer itself – it was a battle to discover the real me.

What if our continual battling with outer circumstances and inner turmoil becomes counterproductive? What if all the worry we feel about so many things in our lives serves no good purpose? What if that worry, doubt, and fear are the very things that are holding us back from being our magnificent selves and living a life of peace and joy?

It's not to suggest that adversity will no longer come knocking. Dealing with adversity is one way we grow. But perhaps there's a better way to work through it than we've ever accessed before.

David Hawkins in "Transcending the Levels of Consciousness" talks about surrender as an integral part of the spiritual path. He recommends 10 simple tools to reveal spiritual truths that have proven their effectiveness over centuries.

The Power of Surrender

"Eagles soar by surrendering to the wind."

A few years ago, I was privileged to watch eagles soar in the skies of Ohio. Of course, it took the effort of their own wings to reach soaring height, but once there, they surrendered to the winds and floated effortlessly.

Surrender does not seem to come easily to humans – at least it hasn't been easy for me. Fiercely independent from a young age, I often separated myself from the support and help that was available for a variety of reasons: unworthiness, lack of trust, or stubborn, egoic pride.

I confess that I don't easily surrender to what I have come to know as a higher power.

It's a bit like planting seeds in your garden that will yield the best carrots ever. You prepare the soil, plant the seeds, cover them with soil, and then water the ground. A week goes by. Your garden shows no sign of anything growing. Another week – still nothing! You can't resist the urge to dig into a tiny patch – just to see what's happening. Of course, when we meddle with Mother Nature's growing cycle, our seeds may not mature and grow into the plants they were intended to be.

So it is with the rhythm and cycles of our universe. Between the time of sewing and reaping there is plenty going on that we can't see. Patience is not my strong suit, so it's hard to resist trying to help the universe along. Each time I interfered though, I noticed it either took longer to manifest my outcome or it was a much more painful process.

If you're a Star Trek fan, you may remember this scene on the bridge of Starship Enterprise. Whenever a new destination was needed, Captain Picard would pick one and then turn to his first officer and say, "Make it so, No. 1." Then I'm guessing he left the bridge for a cup of tea. He didn't hang around to make sure the course was properly charted. He made no suggestions about the route to take. His responsibility was to pick the destination, then surrender the How's and When's to his trusted crew.

I've come to acknowledge that No. 1 on my team is my Higher Self cooperating with that higher consciousness (labeled God, Spirit, Divine Guidance etc.). Once I choose the where or the what, it's Spirit's turn with how to make it happen. Of course, there are some actions that only I can take (such as typing these words) to contribute to the outcome.

My challenge comes in staying focused on my faith and trust in the best outcome possible, even if it might not be the outcome I had originally planned. Sometimes we can't see the perfection of an undesired outcome until we look back.

Tony Robbins says that "life is happening for us, not to us." I've come to believe in this benevolent universe, of which I am an integral part, just as you are an integral part. When we open ourselves to the unknown and the unknowable – when we surrender our ego's need to control every piece, we can reap the highest good that propels us to an even higher level of co-creation.

My main goal these days is to nurture the habit of surrender. It's becoming a more peaceful default!

Death and Dying

Near the beginning of this book, I encouraged you to use the power tools of faith and hope to help you live through and beyond cancer.

But you may now be at the point where you suspect that your body cannot continue. Cancer is here to take you Home. This may or may not scare you and your loved ones.

Our western society does not deal well with the conversation about death and dying, never mind the pending reality. We have this superstitious notion that if we even entertain the idea of death, it brings death closer. But that feels to me like just another form of denial of the situation.

Doctors view death as the enemy – to be fought, sometimes at all costs – as if death were some kind of failure instead of an inevitability for us all.

My personal perspective has changed dramatically since my journey to the afterlife (NDE) in 2007. That experience provided a deep sense of knowing that death of the body is not the end of life.

It's simply a transition to the next grand adventure of our eternal lives as Spirit. This grounding helped enormously when I got cancer. While I don't fear death because of what "heaven" offers, I confess I'm a bit edgy and scared about the process of dying.

While we cannot know what dying is like for us until we experience it, as co-creators with God and the Universe, I believe it would be helpful for us to envision the way we would like to go – quick and painless, an easy surrender, time to bid farewell to loved ones and/or whatever else you envision. Just as we have the power to choose and plan ways to live our lives, could we not also participate in the orchestration of the demise of our bodies? It's a question I don't have the answer for, but what if...?

(**Side Note:** Now here, I'm not talking about assisted death for those with terminal illness, although that is an option where I live in Canada.)

What I do want to state is that even if your days are very limited, you're still in charge. There is help available through religious and spiritual communities to support you and your loved ones through this time.

Use a journal to help you come to terms with issues and/or relationships that are uppermost in your mind. Facing the loss of your life is another level of grieving that only you can take. You may not want to share innermost thoughts with family, so your journal can become a wonderful confidant.

I'm suggesting you get very clear about what's most important to you in your last months, weeks, days, and minutes. If you feel prayer is helpful, then pray to the God of your understanding to help you transition the way you desire.

You may have experienced others who went through their transition from life to afterlife. Death of loved ones is not new to me: my mother died alone very suddenly in hospital of a brain aneurism.

Just days before, she had been diagnosed with leukemia with the prospect of a gradual wasting of her body – not a happy thought for a 40-year-old active, athletic woman. Two of her best friends visited her shortly before she died. To this day, I wish I'd had a chance to say goodbye, and at the same time, I'm so grateful she didn't suffer a lingering death.

My youngest brother, a daredevil who was into extreme sports, lost his life at 23 in a diving accident with only a friend as witness. He was gone in an instant. I hadn't seen him in months, but just two days before he died, he was at my house helping us paint a bathroom. I found out later that he had recently reconnected with all of us that he cared about. I believe he knew, on some other conscious level, that it was his time, so he showed up to have one last visit.

My sister, Monica, who lived in California, was at home under palliative care when her body started shutting down from a ravaging cancer. She had nurses providing 24/7 care to support her. In the last couple of weeks of her life, there was a steady stream of visitors who came to say goodbye, though no one mentioned that it was the reason for their visit.

I flew to be with her for several days before she passed. It was enough to her that I was there. She did not want deep and meaningful conversations, so we kept it light and laughed a lot.

We watched the Summer Olympics, particularly the equestrian events and any other programs that took her fancy. She dozed a lot of the time. She expressed her gratitude for my being there.

Three days after her 50th birthday, she transitioned at home with my younger brother by her side. It was not an easy or peaceful passing – maybe because she fought to stay to the very end.

THE HEALING CALL OF CANCER

We can't know if cancer comes to take us home, so it only makes sense to get as prepared as possible. That saying "prepare for the worst and hope for the best" is appropriate here.

I remember when my grandmother, still in good health in her 70s, hesitantly asked if I would accompany her to the Funeral Home so she could pick out her casket. Off we went. While it seemed strange to be in the funeral home when there was no imminent funeral, it enabled us to ask questions and be curious about how things worked.

At our leisure, we wandered through a room filled with caskets and urns. The funeral representative left us in peace, which allowed us to giggle when I suggested to my grandmother that she climb in the casket of her choice just to make sure it fit. "Look," I said. "I don't want you haunting me because I picked the wrong one!"

Instead of seeming morbid, it became a fond memory. Plus, when it came time to plan her funeral (she was over 87), I was able to guide both her children in decision-making because I had been privy to her wishes.

It seems easier to help an elderly loved one plan for their passing. But when death seems premature, especially for parents of young children, it is much harder.

Before you are too weak to make decisions, I recommend getting your affairs in order.

- Do you have a current will and a personal directive?
- Have you appointed someone with Power of Attorney and/ or an Executor?
- Where are important documents filed such as banking information and account numbers?
- What about passwords for computer files – keys to locked

    cabinets?
- What about palliative care arrangements?
- What about funeral arrangements?

Being prepared in this way will save your loved ones from some anguish and potential court challenges (especially if you have no will) as they settle your estate.

Grief hits everyone differently. Your loved ones may be reluctant to have the kinds of courageous conversations that are necessary. In that case, you may need a friend's help.

In addition to the legal practicalities, consider creating a checklist of things to do or to be done that are important to you. For example, have you left anything heartfelt unsaid to loved ones?

Months before her diagnosis when she felt something was wrong, my mom sorted through family pictures and created photo albums for each of us four kids. I remember it taking her hours and hours. Having those was a great comfort when she passed.

A friend who cared for her invalid husband helped him in his last days record a goodbye video for each of his children. Tribute and gratitude letters can be especially precious to our loved ones, as can the sound of a loved one's voice. Bless technology for the many options available these days.

If you live in your own home, you may also decide to give prized possessions to your family early and/or clear out any clutter. I dislike the idea of leaving a mess for my kids, so I've downsized considerably over the years. I admit I was a bit taken aback when one woman, a bit of a pack rat, blithely said she wasn't throwing anything away. "My children will just have to deal with it."

Having been an estate executor, I know how much work it is, even when the person leaves very little behind. Remember though, you can only do what you can do. Ask friends to help. They won't be as emotionally attached to your stuff as you or your kids might be.

While your struggles will be over when you pass, the struggles of your loved ones will start in a different way. Of course, you are **not** responsible for how they will handle your passing, but you can help ease their suffering by keeping the lines of communication open.

I remember when I was being wheeled into surgery in 2007, I had this thought that this could be the end of me. Immediately, my son came to mind, and I felt regret that I wouldn't get to say goodbye.

Because it wasn't my time, I've invested precious moments since then making sure he knows how much I love him. And I've been getting my affairs and my household in order.

Assisted Dying

Before I move on from thoughts on death and dying, I wanted to share the little I know about assisted dying for the terminally ill. It's legal here in Canada and I believe in some of the states in the U.S. No one makes this decision without a great deal of thought.

I know two couples personally whose loved ones chose this route. In my province, you must be of sound mind to choose this (no one can choose for you) plus you need an examination and signatures from three different doctors. You are free to stop the process and change your mind at any point.

One person I knew was a young woman with ALS in her 40s whose health had deteriorated to the point where a horrific death was all that was left. She was not willing to suffer like that, nor did she want her children and family to experience her last days in that way.

In the second family, an elderly father knew his health was failing. His aging wife was suffering from dementia. He had no desire to end up alone in a nursing home existing on machines and dependent on nursing staff. While he was still of sound mind, he followed the legal process and picked the day of his passing.

In every case I've heard about, although it was a choice that shocked each family at the outset, the peaceful passing was a relief to loved ones.

Will we suffer the hell of eternal damnation if this is what we choose? I have no idea. Despite biblical references, I doubt that any human knows for sure, so I leave any judging about this kind of issue to God.

I can't help but wonder, though, why we provide a painless passing to aging or suffering pets, yet we feel squeamish about this option for a loved one dealing with a terminal condition.

This is another one of those courageous conversations that can arise to help us deal with casting off our bodies in a way that serves us emotionally, mentally, and spiritually.

Afterword

Your Cancer Story – What Legacy will You Leave?

Somehow, I knew that documenting my cancer journey was important, so I started writing about the events and my thoughts and feelings soon after the diagnosis. Initially I wrote to come to terms with the horror I was going through.

To know that something is eating away inside of you that you feel helpless to battle or overcome is its own brand of terror. But putting it down on paper took it out of my mind and eventually helped me cope as I sought to understand why I went through what I did.

Despite being surrounded by staunch supporters, much of this experience is lived alone by the sufferer. My journal became my audience when I was in pain or felt hopeless and helpless.

The suffering I experienced eventually seeded the ground of my new purpose and destiny. This book and my previous one "Magnificent Misery – From Adversity to Ecstasy" have become part of that new direction for me.

While you may have no intention of writing a book, let me emphasize that some form of sharing is helpful for the healing of everyone involved. There are many ways of sharing that last long after we're gone. For example:

1. Heartfelt letters to loved ones that tell them what they've meant to you and what you hope for them.
2. Videos or written experiences with your children to provide future comfort.
3. Relationship-mending; this is a time to forgive and ask for forgiveness.

4. Recorded interviews – enlist the help of a friend to create a series of heartfelt questions that you can answer.

Regardless of your method and the amount you share, your experience holds meaning for you, even if you don't know it now. Your experience will have meaning for others, too, that can add to their lives in ways you can't possibly imagine. Share who you are, my magnificent friend. We will all be better for that sharing.

Phoenix

by Sue Paulson ©

Burned to ashes
Life blown away,
I sit in emptiness.
Lost, searching, alone.

All that mattered
matters not, anymore.
I wait,
cry into the silence.
Mourn the old.
Time passes.

Pin feathers
of new wonderings
emerge.

Flickers of light
dance behind closed eyelids.
Rosy gold & flames of violet
beckon me home.

My heart opens to
new feelings,
pink skin,
the breath of life,
love, tenderness,
meaning.

I grow and grow
to be
ME
Awash in Ecstasy.
Phoenix Risen.

In Conclusion

It has been such a privilege to share with you, not only this slice of my healing journey, but my thoughts and ideas for you on your journey.

As I said earlier, take what resonates with and serves you and leave the rest. My fondest desire is that *The Healing Call of Cancer* has provided support and inspiration for you and your family.

May you grow and heal magnificently through your cancer journey. One day, perhaps we'll meet on the Other Side and share stories of triumphs and victories. Blessings to all!

Sue

Books that Helped Sue to Grow

(In Alphabetical Order)

1. *A Better Normal – Your Guide to Rediscovering Intimacy after Cancer* by Tess Deveze
2. *A Thousand Names for Joy – Living in Harmony with the Way Things Are*, Byron Katie with Stephen Mitchell
3. *Communion with God,* by Neale Donald Walsch
4. *Illusions – The Adventures of a Reluctant Messiah,* by Richard Bach
5. *Loving What Is,* Byron Katie
6. *One,* by Richard Bach
7. *The Body Keeps the Score,* Bessel A. Van Kolk M.D.
8. *The Myth of Normal,* Gabor Mate M.D.
9. *The Way of Mastery* by Shanti Christo Foundation
10. *Transcending the Levels of Consciousness – The Stairway to Enlightenment,* by David R Hawkins, M.D., Ph.D.
11. *When the Body Says No – The Cost of Hidden Stress* by Gabor Mate
12. *Your Body's Telling You: Love Yourself!* By Lise Bourbeau

The Journey Continues...

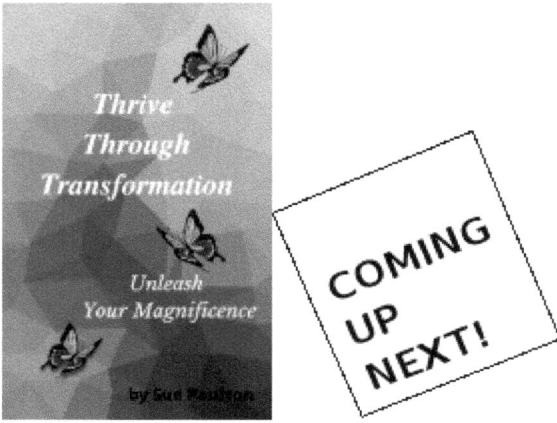

Join Sue as she inspires us to move through our adversities and resulting fears to the life we deserve – Heaven on Earth. How do we awaken to and embrace the magnificence we are? How do we practically apply that magnificence?

Until   then,   check   out   Sue's   memoir:

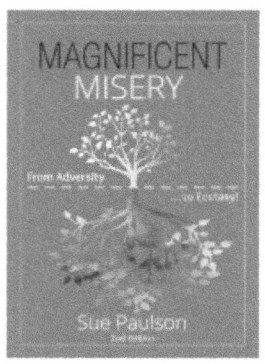

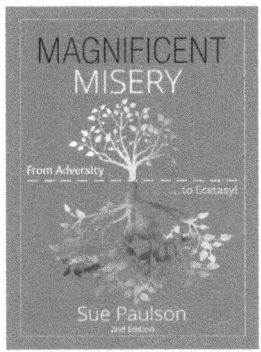

About the Author

Sue Paulson

Despite her knocking knees, Sue recited a poem at church and reveled in her first audience applause at age 10. Drawn to the front of the room, she started teaching a personal growth program in her late 20s. She moved on to create and conduct corporate workshops throughout Alberta with topics such as stress reduction, conflict resolution, and team development.

A self-taught educator, Sue began the first of her 15 years of part time teaching at MacEwan University in 1996. Her topics - business writing, public speaking, and study skills.

In 1999 she published her first best-selling book, *Tips & Tools for Student Success*. It was followed in 2003 by her award-winning *Tips & Tools to Speak with Confidence – Keys to Finding Your Voice*.

Thriving since her near-death experience in 2007 and bouts of cancer in 2011 and 2012, Sue published her best-selling memoir *Magnificent Misery – From Adversity to Ecstasy* in 2015 and launched the second edition in 2022.

In 2023, she co-founded the Magnificence Lab – an online community for budding Magnificence Mentors.

https://magnificencelab.org

Her passion - inspiring others to Be their magnificent selves in order to create heaven on earth.

Want more from Sue? Subscribe to her Sue Paulson YouTube channel and watch her videos:

- Heaven on Earth

videos designed to inspire you to continue creating your Heaven on Earth

- Tea with Sue

104 videos about what life is teaching Sue.

- Magnificence Moments

Short Videos - remove blocks & unlock your magnificence.

- Healing Call of Cancer

Videos designed to provide cancer sufferers and their families with information and hope

To Book Sue as Your Next Inspirational Speaker, visit her website:
https://suepaulson.com

or e-mail her: sue@suepaulson.com

Her Topics Include:

- The Magnificence Matrix
- The Healing Call of Cancer
- Creating Your Brand of Heaven on Earth
- Pathways to Magnificence

Don't miss out!

Visit the website below and you can sign up to receive emails whenever Sue Paulson publishes a new book. There's no charge and no obligation.

https://books2read.com/r/B-A-NRDX-MKQZE

BOOKS 2 READ

Connecting independent readers to independent writers.

Also by Sue Paulson

Magnificent Misery - From Adversity to Ecstasy
The Healing Call of Cancer

Watch for more at https://suepaulson.com.

Milton Keynes UK
Ingram Content Group UK Ltd.
UKHW032317121024
449481UK00012B/441